Everything I Wish I Could Tell You

A Guide for the Most Dangerous Journey

THOMAS REED

Everything I Wish I Could Tell You
Copyright © 2023 by Thomas Reed

All rights reserved. No part of this publication may be reproduced, distributed, or transmitted in any form or by any means, including photocopying, recording, or other electronic or mechanical methods, without the prior written permission of the author, except in the case of brief quotations embodied in critical reviews and certain other non-commercial uses permitted by copyright law.

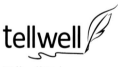

Tellwell Talent
www.tellwell.ca

ISBN
978-0-2288-9515-2 (Paperback)

To those unsure what the controls are, let the lessons I've been through guide yours.

Who compels you to judge? If it is your wish—you must prove first that you are capable of justice. As judges, you must stand higher than that which is to be judged: as it is, you have only come later. The guests that come last to the table should rightly take the last places: and will you take the first? Then do some great and mighty deed: the place may be prepared for you then, even though you do come last.

Friedrich Nietzsche

We are the smith, the swordsman, and the sword.

Temper your mind so that it cuts swiftly.

The weight of the handle must be balanced with the blade.

A blade doesn't remain sharp without care.

The swordsman cannot swing confidently without practice.

PROLOGUE

If you would think of this book as a lighthouse in the dark, warning passersby of rocks so not to become stranded on the shore.

Survive; everything else comes afterwards. If you are lost, if you are looking for a reason, the only one you will find here is this, survive. You are already doing it partially when you wake up every day and you go to sleep every night.

The next step is to take accountability of that, and to turn survival into thriving. To make the most of your time. Choosing to live, and just continuing to live are two very different things. The actions you take every day make up the space between them.

You may not like everything you have to do, but there are always things that you must do. If you intend to choose survival, if you choose to wake up every day, to live actively within your life, then there is only one way to do that.

With that out of the way, onto everything else that comes afterwards.

GETTING STARTED—NOTHING TO LOSE

Your life belongs to you. Your memories, your talents, your skills, and your dreams. Live your life in a way that no matter what happens, you can still count on yourself. Every day you wake up is a victory. Turn yourself into someone who could survive the world ending.

I do not assume to know or understand the life of anyone else. I will never know what it is like to live your life. I will never know the emotions you feel; how could I ever do that? The only person's eyes I have ever seen through are my own.

These lessons that I offer to you are what my life has taught me. You may have lived through these lessons already. Or you may not have yet. If you haven't yet I offer this book as a guide, and a hand to hold onto. You are going to be fine; this too will pass, tomorrow will come, and the sun will shine again.

A basic idea, a basic question can change a life.

Food for thought—What has life taught you?

SELF-REFLECTION AND MEDITATION

You need to practice self-reflection. To be able to learn from our lives, we need to be able to examine our lives. This means recognizing that we are not just our emotions, we are not just our intentions, and we are not just our impulses.

When we allow our thoughts to wander and to drift through our consciousness, we need to pay attention to what thoughts make us want to become distracted. Often, we will do things to stop ourselves from thinking about the things that we really should be coming to terms with. This could be an awkward interaction with a co-worker, or something that we regret doing or thinking. The more we avoid thinking about it, the more it will keep coming back to haunt us. Instead, sit down with the thought and ask yourself what you learned from it. Then dismiss it and move past it.

So how do you step away from your thoughts? How do you separate yourself so that you can understand what it is you are feeling? How do you even feel emotions? You are probably used to feeling angry, feeling sad, and feeling happy. But your entire existence isn't about being angry, sad, or happy. As if the entire human existence could be contained within those simple names. Your emotions are a part of you, but they do not make up your entire existence.

Your goal is to recognize how these emotions feel. Do you feel a tightness in your chest? Maybe your head feels heavy? How fast is your heart beating? There is little I can do to guide you in recognizing your emotions with these words. But you can never hope to control something that you cannot even recognize. The only way to recognize them is to experience them.

I can only offer this suggestion to help you learn to control your emotions. The next time your emotions overcome you, take a step back, take a deep breath, close your eyes, and take an inventory of how you are feeling. What does your body feel? We're not robots. Our emotions will make themselves known, but just remember that you are more than them.

Until we learn the lessons, we are doomed to repeat our lessons throughout our lives.

To put it simply, if we keep making a mistake, we will continue to make that mistake until we learn why it is a mistake.

Food for thought—When you sit down and just think, what comes to mind?

SLEEP RENEWS YOUR BODY

Regular sleeping habits will ensure we get enough rest to consistently go into each day at our best. As well, by maintaining a regular sleeping habit we will sleep easier. There are a few ways to make sure that when we lay down to sleep, we will fall asleep easier.

Chief among them is to stop using your bed for everything.

Our brain thinks that whatever we do in bed is what we are supposed to be doing in bed.

If we use our phone in bed, we will want to use it more.

If we watch shows in bed, we will want to watch more of them.

If we eat in bed, our brain will tell us it is time to eat.

If we practice activities in bed, we will want to do those.

If the only thing we do in bed is sleep, our brain will tell us it is time to sleep.

Another main factor is how much energy we expend in a day. How close are we pushing ourselves to our limit? It isn't a great mystery that if we spend all day exerting ourselves, working out, and staying active that we will sleep easier at night. The same is true for mental exhaustion. If we are having difficulty sleeping at night, it may be that we aren't pushing ourselves hard enough mentally.

Getting control of our sleep schedule and turning it into something consistent should be our main priority. A proper night's sleep is crucial to be able to make decisions on a higher level. Not getting enough sleep will not only change how you act, but it will make tasks more difficult. It will make keeping your focus harder, and it will be harder to remember what you are being told.

Food for thought—What am I doing immediately prior to trying to sleep?

ASSIGN PURPOSE TO YOUR LIFE

You will find your own purpose in life. This piece of advice permeates everything in life, but without anyone going into detail on how to do this. So, let's go into detail. What I suggest is assigning purpose to the pieces of our life, which when put together create the whole. Typically, the best way to build anything is to start small and go from there. So, what's the first step to take?

Our life is made up of thousands upon thousands of tiny pieces that we take for granted as being a part of our life. Assigning purpose to the smaller details of our life will give us clarity on the broader whole.

This action is about organizing our life in a way that it fits into our life. Everyone finds their own way to thrive, and their own way to make things work in this crazy world. Some need a perfectly sorted and labelled existence, with not a hair out of place. Some live for the mess, somehow remembering that their green pen is in the pocket of a jacket they wore three days ago. Organizing doesn't look the same for everyone. The nerds among us understand this fact already, even if they don't implement it in their day-to-day lives. How you organize something can be deeply personal. Organizing is about being efficient, and it's about making your life easier.

Bubble sort, selections sort, merge sort, and quick sort.

Even some of the most organized only do it in a certain way because that's how they were shown. For the sake of an argument, let's borrow the idea of labelling, and apply it to more than just files in a folder. When you think of your life, do you label different parts of it? If you started to break up your day, your life, labelling each piece of it, and assigning purpose to it, what would it look like?

Let's keep it simple, though there is plenty of room to make it more complicated if that is what will help you.

Your life looks like this when we sort it into pieces.

Rest	Sleep	Leisure	Reflect
Effort	Develop	Maintain	

Effort—Develop
The idea here is the times in your day where you are actively increasing your abilities. Pushing yourself to learn new things or in some way to grow past where you are now. This is true in a social sense as well as a personal sense. It is wide ranging, from developing your physical abilities by playing a sport, to developing your mental state by practising algebra.

Effort—Maintain
This is exactly as it sounds. It's the status quo. It's not pushing yourself, and it's just doing what needs to be done to maintain a part of your life. It's cooking rice for dinner instead of trying a new recipe. It's doing laundry. Basically, it's the work you do that doesn't challenge you to be more than you are.

Rest—Reflect
Reflection is the time you spend with your thoughts, thinking about your day, and thinking about what is to come. It's thinking about what you have already done, your past and how that will inform your actions in the future. It's asking yourself how you would react differently next time.

Rest—Leisure
Leisure is the time you spend not developing new skills, not maintaining your life, and not reflecting. It could be watching shows, or mindlessly scrolling through social media. Leisure in this case is the things you do that don't take effort, and don't offer a chance to reflect.

Food for thought—When you write down thoughts about your typical day, how much of it now has purpose?

YOUR BALANCE IS TELLING

Learning to balance is one of the first things we do as children. To learn to walk we must first learn to crawl. Our balance is something we can always refine, and sure, at a certain point we'll see diminishing returns. But finding balance in every aspect of your life means so much more than just your physical balance.

How does someone who spends their day in an office on a computer find balance? That's hardly the only facet of their lives, and so balance for them becomes what they do outside of their work. Balance is part of our physical and mental health; it helps to keep us grounded when the world feels unstable. It's one of the easiest things for us to refine. It takes no tools; it takes no special instruction. All it takes is a desire to improve it. Some may argue the opposite, that balance is hard to refine, but when combined with organization, what is out of balance will make itself apparent. The great thing about balance is that when you're leaning too far to one side other aspects will suffer, and so all it takes to recognize when you're out of balance is looking for what is falling apart.

We don't need to be a master to benefit from having better balance. Even just a small win will make every day a little easier. Better balance is a tool to navigate life; to be able to move past obstacles that would hinder others. It means catching ourselves before we fall. It means that when we do fall, we are able to get back up. It means being able to stand our ground even if the ground is moving. It means recognizing when we're losing our balance and being able to adjust for it.

If we were to imagine the entire world as living on a see-saw, there would be some of us living on either side, and there would be some of us walking the middle. Those on either side would have their counters, and those in the middle walking the line would be careful about how much weight they would be placing on either side of the beam.

Food for thought—A fall can take many forms, from a physical fall to emotional distress, to a social issue. What is out of balance in your life right now?

YOU NEVER KNOW WHAT YOU'LL LEARN NEXT

The biggest strength of anyone who can keep an open mind is their ability to learn from everything. Pick and choose what you pay attention to because that is what you'll remember. Of course, there is such a plethora of options put in front of us that even just picking something can be daunting. The more often we go out into the world with the intention of learning something, the more often we will learn something.

Too often we get caught up in our emotions to be able to learn something from the big flashy events in our lives. If we do learn, it's usually in the form of fear depending on how things went. Gaining a new fear isn't hard, but that's hardly the only thing you can learn. Are you a passive observer or an active observer? Are you someone who believes in being a lifelong learner? Isn't the key to that goal the ability to learn from life?

There are countless pieces of information being thrown at us every single day, and most of it we tune out. It's completely unrealistic to expect us to remember all of it. Do you really need to remember the price of a spice you buy only once every five years? That sounds like a quick way to getting information overload if you try and absorb every little thing in your life. Instead, it might serve us better to just try to remain an active participant in our lives. One of the simplest ways to do this is to keep track of what we learn; or in other words, journaling, and note taking.

Maybe we'll learn where a crow roosts, or maybe we'll learn a life lesson. Not everything we learn is important for our everyday life; it's more about being consistent and practising it as a skill. The more often we go about life looking for things to learn, the more we will learn.

Surprise, surprise. If we do something more often, we get better at it.

Food for thought—What did you learn yesterday?

WHAT YOU PUT INTO THIS WORLD

Too few people take proper care to monitor their impact on the world around them. Often, they are completely ignorant of it. They walk through life as if they are on a path that they hold no sway over. Their mind forever in the clouds, simply moving from one point to another. Dreaming of a better life while forgetting to live the one they are already living. Each day is indistinguishable from the last, each month simply marked by a calendar, and the years blending together. One day they will find themselves on their deathbed asking, "What did I do?" They spent it dreaming. They lived their entire life without taking ownership of the choices they made every single day.

The good news is you are here, you are reading this, and you are already on the path to recognizing the choices you make. Being aware of our impact on the world and being aware of our life is the same thing. So how do we recognize the impact we have on the world? Like habits, like building anything, you start small, and you start with the first brick.

The biggest delusion any of us have is that the world revolves around us, and yet we can't imagine anything that we do that has any effect on the world. This is completely ridiculous. It doesn't matter what we do, but what we do shapes the world. Because the actions of one influence the actions of those around them. If we have the ability to make a choice, everything we choose to do is important.

We never know who is watching. Some kid watched you pick up trash and put it in the trash can, and now they think that's cool because someone else did it. Maybe you say thank you when getting off the bus, and so those around you also say thank you. If you are someone who is confident enough to make a choice, you will never know who is watching you and might take what you do as something they should do.

It's a disservice to yourself to think you are so unimportant that what you do doesn't matter. Though on the flip side it doesn't matter. You're still just one person, one life, one perspective. But look at the world as if it's a mirror reflection of you. It's just one mirror multiplied by every single person on earth. Do you like what you see when you look at your life? What if every single person on the planet was living your life, would you be happy in that world?

It's bigger than you, but it starts with you.

You want to be part of something bigger than yourself? Congratulations, you already are. Often, we have trouble removing ourselves from the picture and zooming out. We get obsessed with the idea that if the world doesn't know our name, then we aren't a part of the world. That could not be further from the truth. Each person contributes to the glorious, ordered chaos that is our world. Every action you take radiates through your life, touching and weaving a little bit of you into the lives of others.

Food for thought—How quiet the forest would be if only the most beautiful bird sang.

ONE IS INFINITELY BIGGER THAN ZERO

This may sound completely obvious, and really it is, but for some reason when we are laying on the couch wondering what to do, how often do we choose "nothing?" There are people who spend their entire lives waiting for "something" to happen, and then when something does happen, they are upset it didn't turn out the way they expected. These are the same people who will complain about being bored, and who will say there is nothing to do. The world is full of these people, who will ride the waves of events. Place no thought to the comings and goings of these people. They are not living your life, and their participation is not required for you to live yours. If you were to base your life on them, you would never have direction because each and every one of them would point a different way.

You are an action taker; you know that even one action per day is three hundred and sixty-five actions per year. You are a decision maker, someone who chooses to make a choice. We've all heard it before. "The journey of one thousand miles begins with a single step." Before we can get to the thousandth mile, we must go through all those that came before it. Before we get good at something, we must be bad at something. Just the fact that you choose to do something, anything, puts you ahead of where you were before. If you don't know what the next step is to do something, you aren't thinking small enough. Break it down into as small of steps as you need to, to be able to understand what needs to happen next.

Anything worth doing, is worth doing badly.

One is infinitely bigger than zero.

If we want to get into better shape, there is only one way to do that.

If we want to learn more languages, there is only one way to do that.

If we want to meet more people, there is only one way to do that.

Ask anyone who is a regular at a gym and they can tell you that you don't get swole after one work out. It takes dedication, and it takes regular, consistent effort. The same is true for every aspect of our lives. You put in zero effort, and you will get the same back in results. The more effort we put in per day, the faster we will see results. It's up to you to determine what you can sustain consistently.

For example, if you are trying to become a tidier person, set an alarm ten minutes per day, every day just for cleaning. The important part here is consistency. You will find that by committing to something even as small as 0.007% of your day, every day that your entire life will start to shift just by that one small commitment you made to yourself.

The same is true for anything we set our mind to do on a regular basis. The biggest super power we have is compound interest, and that is true for real life as much as it is true for our financial life. So, compound those activities, stay active, keep your mind fresh, and make decisions actively to always be choosing one over zero.

Food for thought—Do you have twenty minutes a day to live a better life?

A WIN IS A WIN NO MATTER HOW SMALL

Too often we focus solely on the big tasks, basing our internal value on the outcomes of a few big things in life. In reality, each big success is made up of thousands of tiny wins all rolled up together. These small wins often go completely unrecognized as part of the path to achieving an overall goal. But the reality is without them, we never would have made it to the end.

What do these small, tiny, yet crucial wins look like?

It's the little things we do every day.

It's getting out of bed.

It's brushing our teeth, having a shower.

It's the attitude we bring into each day.

It's keeping track of our progress.

It's always doing what we can to make tomorrow's life easier.

It's offering a hand to someone who needs a hand.

These aren't things on their own that are worth celebrating, but they add up quickly when we stay on top of them every day. By staying aware of these small wins, we also allow ourselves to be critical of our lessons. This is part of always moving forward in life. Every win is a step forward, and by treating every loss as a lesson, it can turn even our losses into a step forward into our future.

It's in this way we become invincible. By learning from our mistakes, we maintain our ability to look toward the future and not spend all our time regretting the past. So, allow our lives to be our teacher. Our future will always come, and there will always be more wins to be had.

Food for thought—What small wins have you had today?

OWN YOUR MIND—RECOGNIZE A CHOICE

One of the biggest steps we take on our path to maturity is learning to take accountability for our actions. That is all well and good to say, but if we don't even recognize some of our actions as choices in the first place it can be hard to see them as something to take accountability for. Often, we are not even aware of the choices we make, or rather that they are even choices. Every single day we make hundreds, if not thousands of choices. Most of them would be viewed as inconsequential if thought of as one-time events. No matter the choices you make, no matter how small, their cumulative nature will build up over time with the result being the life you are living right now.

No matter how mundane, or how chaotic your life is, it is the product of the choices you have made up to this point. Coincidences and the choices of others will have influence on your life, but ultimately you determine the shape of your life. Depending upon where you are at in your life, you will either find yourself agreeing with this statement or not.

Ten years ago, if you had decided to start practising a new language every day how fluent would you be now?

Five years ago, if you had decided to start working out every day what shape would you be in right now?

In five years, starting now, what level of shape will you be in?

In ten years starting now, what are you going to be an expert in?

Make the choice to grow, and you will.

There are choices that will help you, and choices that will hurt you. All the same they are choices. The consequences of your actions are what happen when you make a choice. Some consequences will make themselves apparent, and some will not. Everything little thing you do will affect your life and the lives of others because what you do is your life.

Food for thought—How many choices do you make in a day?

A PATTERN IS NOT LIMITED TO ART

We can't see the forest from the trees, but that doesn't stop us from knowing we're inside a forest. If we are no more than beasts, following our impulses to find our next meal, would we be able to recognize that we're in a forest? If we stood in the middle of a city, the horizon blocked by buildings that reach to the skies, would we recognize we're inside a city? How would we go about identifying what city we're in if no one told you?

This same rationale can be extended to the patterns of life. We may not know which patterns we're a part of, where our piece lies, but all the same, our piece exists. The universe is chaotic. Just as a forest can burn to the ground, a city can fall into ruin, and a pattern can end. Just because we are part of a pattern does not mean it must repeat. It simply takes a rogue piece, a pebble in the road to throw a cart off course. Whatever pattern emerges from that new course will have its own pieces.

Our actions, our choices, our lives are part of a pattern that is larger than any of us forest dwellers can recognize. So, I ask, fellow forest dweller, what patterns are you part of? What patterns form in your life? A pattern, a repeating situation, a common mistake can sometimes be so mundane you don't even notice it.

Your place in the larger patterns of life is guaranteed. It is your birthright, as it is for all of us. Spend some time thinking about the smaller patterns that exist in your life, and you'll find where you need to make changes. After that, making the changes is up to you.

Food for thought—What patterns do you find beautiful?

BEING HONEST WITH OURSELVES

One of the hardest obstacles we face in life sounds like something that should be easy to overcome. Maybe it is for some, but that's certainly not the case for all. All it is, is accepting ourselves for who we are right now in this moment. It means recognizing our flaws for what they are, and it means knowing what our strengths are. It also means recognizing when we are lying to ourselves. It happens more often than one might think. We push aside a thought because we don't know if we should trust the thought or trust what we were told. We ignore parts of ourselves out of fear. We don't even take the time to consider them for fear of not being able to turn them away once we do allow ourselves to think on those thoughts.

Being honest with ourselves is as much about learning to trust ourselves, as it is learning to control ourselves. It's being able to identify those intrusive thoughts and performing a pro and con list in our head about whether they are helpful or harmful. If we never even interact with those thoughts, then in moments of weakness, when we're emotional, stressed, and distraught, we're more likely to give in to something we would otherwise never do. It's in this way that we're looking for balance within our own mind.

It's about coming to terms with our desires, but not allowing our desires to deceive us. What would you prefer in life? Someone who asks you for what they want up front, or someone who sneaks around back to take what they want from you? So, why not encourage your own subconscious to be upfront about what it is that you want.

You need to find your own conclusions here because this is only a guide. Being honest with myself means I'm not trying to create a clone who thinks the same as me but someone who shines in their own brilliant colours.

Food for thought—What are you not saying out loud?

DELAYED GRATIFICATION

Acquired tastes generally have the best flavours. It's often the case that at first, the taste can be overwhelming, bitter, or in some cases underwhelming. Once we acquire a taste for it, delayed gratification is the sweetest nectar life has to offer.

The unfortunate reality of the world now is it feeds us instant gratification by a tube. While sweet, it comes as soon as we want it, but the costs are disguised and shrouded. We have it at our fingertips in most cases, always within reach. We can seek whatever form we want with relative ease. The biggest danger of instant gratification is the hidden costs, the fees. They will come due, and they will get paid in some form or another. With delayed gratification you sow all the costs up front and reap the rewards at harvest.

Delayed gratification is much more about recognizing the benefits that lay in the journey to completion rather than the final reward that falls at the goal post. It's about taking advantage of the skills we sharpen while completing a task. It's about knowing that once we complete something, it stays complete. Throughout life we will be presented with many different forms of shortcuts to reach whatever goal. Some will be a quick cut through, and others will be alleyways. Some alleyways will be dangerous, and some won't. Sometimes what looks like a shortcut will end up taking longer than if we had remained on our path.

Food for thought—What skill did you develop in your last project?

If you were to need an example of the costs of choosing instant over delayed gratification, we only need to look at the food we eat every single day. Let's say you choose the instant option for breakfast, lunch, and dinner. You eat cereal for breakfast, canned soup for lunch, and frozen pizza for dinner. Sure, the costs may seem obvious. You paid someone else for prepackaged, easy to eat meals, and you saved on time spent preparing them. Already I know you are thinking about the hidden costs, but I'll run you through them.

Hidden cost number one: the cost of opportunity. Every single time you opt to allow someone else to prepare a meal for you, you lose the opportunity to refine your own cooking skills. Refining your cooking skills increases your own skill set and ability to look after yourself.

Hidden cost number two: the cost of nutrition. The nutrients provided in the above meals are limited in scope, and do not give you significant room to adjust for weaknesses in your diet. In meals you prepare yourself, you have more freedom to add or remove things depending on what is best for you.

Sometimes it's worth it, sometimes it's not. It's much more important that we are actively thinking about what hidden costs our impulses will leave us with. They are not all as obvious as what foods we eat. Hyper vigilance isn't going to do us any good either. It will just leave you paranoid and unable to enjoy the splendours of life. It would be better to suggest asking if the shortcut is a bad deal or not.

Food for thought—What instant gratification left you with a regret?

ASK YOURSELF WHY

Why did you write that?
Why did you talk to that person?
Why did you say what you said?
Why did you do that thing?
Why did you go to that place?
Why did you buy that one?
Why did you dress that way?
Why are you wearing those shoes?
Why are you working that job?
Why did you wake up?

BE HARSH ON YOURSELF, GENTLE WITH OTHERS

Don't make it your job to give someone else a reality check. Not only will you not be thanked for it, but you may also be resented for it. The only person we should be concerned about keeping in check with reality is ourselves. Everyone is going to go through different things in life, and many of us will learn lessons from just living life. There are things that we can never understand until we go through it ourselves. It's in this way that this book is only a reflection of the life that's been playing out in front of my eyes.

No one will ever fully understand you. No one will ever fully know your intentions. No one will ever fully know your limits. Except for you. You are the only one whose been there the whole time. You are the only one whose seen life through your eyes. You are the only one who makes you walk forward into every day. That's not to say what others have to say isn't valuable, just that they too have only ever seen life through their own eyes.

So, if we are the one with the greatest understanding of our actions, we should also be the most critical of them. Just as our muscles grow by being torn and stressed, you need to tear apart your motivations, your actions, and your life, so that you can build it up bigger than it ever was. Destruction for the sake of itself is a waste. It's more about assessing the position you're in and finding what needs work.

It's not your job to do that for anyone else, just like no one can go to the gym for another. No one can force someone to grow that doesn't want to. If we want to see those around us shine the brightest, then we must shine as brilliantly as we can, so things don't appear as dark and treacherous as they once did. Find a way to use your light to nourish others. Make growth attractive, so that those around you will reach for their own great heights.

Food for thought—After you're done being upset with yourself, don't forget to forgive yourself.

SAYING NO TO YOURSELF

The entire world is full of people trying to change the world. The only world any one of us really has any level of control over is ourselves, everything else is waves. If we don't practice control over ourselves, then what hope do we have of understanding the actions we take? What this is really about is self-control and being able to tell ourselves no when we need to. About being able to stay consistent in the actions we take. And being able to know how we will react before we must.

Like every other skill we develop in life, self-control is one that if we don't practice, we will not develop. Our impulses, our desires, our instincts will lead us, but these motivators are generally only concerned about our immediate future. They will keep us alive in an emergency, but if we live our daily lives relying on instinct and impulses to make our decisions for us, we would be surrendering one of the greatest strengths we have as humans.

Think about what unhealthy habits you have right now. What would be harder? Breaking that unhealthy habit or starting a new healthier habit? How hard is it for you to deny your own impulses to do things? This isn't about denying yourself any pleasures in life, but having the consciousness to choose when and where you allow yourself to give in to impulse. Instinct and impulse are a part of us, but that's it. They are only a part of us, and we shouldn't allow them to fully control our life.

Food for thought—What is one habit that you would stop today if magic existed? How could you stop that habit without magic?

FEAR IS A SIGNAL—NOT AN ACTION

Beyond facing our fears and walking head first into them, there isn't really much we can do to control fear. What we can control is our body, and how we react to something. Unfortunately, I have some bad news for you. To control how you react to a signal you first must learn what that signal feels like. What good will it do if every time you get scared you run away or freeze up?

The only advice I can offer you when learning what that signal feels like is this. Don't forget to breathe as you learn how to control your responses and reactions.

Regulate your breathing and go from there.

> Be wary of those,
> The righteous
> Who hold their heads high,
> No longer meeting your gaze.

The father
Who stood tall,
No longer a hero to anyone.
The dreamer
Who lives in the clouds,
No longer looks to the sky.
The dedicated
Who worked tirelessly,
No longer have a goal.

Food for thought—What fear are you too scared to face?

PROCRASTINATION, AVOIDANCE, AND DISTRACTION

Often, we find the things that we keep putting to the side are the things that we should be doing first. Depending on what it is that we need to do, we may find it just feels too difficult. The more time you have to get something done, the better quality you can create. The more difficult something is, the more important it is to use that time to make a consistent effort on it.

Perhaps it's a longer project that we started with inspiration or enthusiasm, but as it starts taking longer to do, we begin to doubt ourselves. Inspiration is great for getting the ball rolling, but if we intend to produce something we are content with, we need dedication and consistency. When we are inspired, doing whatever it is that is required feels like the most natural thing in the world. If only inspiration could hold our hand the entire way through. But it seems like no matter what it is we put in front of ourselves, eventually we will come to find reasons to look elsewhere for distractions.

Dedication, consistency, and focus are our allies, and it requires practice to keep procrastination, avoidance, and distraction at bay. It's important to be able to tell ourselves that we need to get something done to keep us motivated and on track. Sometimes it's important to force ourselves to just do something, even if we don't want to. It's important to be able to stay on task and focused so that we make progress. When we are staring at something that we know we need to do, but anything and everything seems like a better alternative there's a good chance that the delayed task is something that we should be doing. Often, we would be better served in telling ourselves to tackle it in chunks.

Even the biggest project is made up of a bunch of smaller parts. Viewing the task in smaller chunks can make it seem less daunting. So, identify those individual parts and do them. No one ever builds a castle from the top down; we always start at the base. Build the foundation first by placing one brick at a time. Then, focus on just placing the next brick in the chain and so on. Before you know it, the task will be accomplished.

Food for thought—What single brick can you lay in your next project?

THE ADDICTION TO STANDING YOUR GROUND

Most of us go through this phase initially as children. We all learn of our ability to say no. We learn that we can exert a tiny amount of control on the world around us by refusing to act. Of course, we will experience a varying amount of pushback from the world around us, but the only person we have true control over is ourselves. It can be easy to take this power for granted. To think that it is a skeleton key to life will put you in a spot where you're relying on it, and it doesn't work. But if you don't understand the cost associated with the refusal, even if we get our way it may be a genie's wish and not turn out how we expect it to. For all you know, it could be a missed opportunity, which you will never see again.

For example, you're more than welcome to refuse to exercise. Instead, all that time you could have spent taking care of your body is spent on a couch watching the lives of others. You get your way because you didn't spend time doing something you didn't want to do. Instead, you get to relax on the couch. It's a win-win, right? If you believe that, well I'll let you believe that's a win. You certainly seem to.

You're also more than welcome to refuse to eat what is offered, but you might regret that decision. Especially if that food is not offered a second time.

Additionally, anytime you are reliant upon the actions of others, your ability to refuse, your ability to say no, loses a lot of its power. So, respect its power, but do not overestimate it. It may be better to view the ability of standing your ground as a negotiation. Be prepared to redraw the lines in the sand or be prepared to walk away along with all the consequences that will follow. We must learn for ourselves what we can and cannot walk away from, but if it's the only water in a desert, do we really have a choice?

Standing your ground is a powerful action. But holding onto your power in some cases can result in you making enemies. Perhaps when you didn't really need to be making enemies. This action can in turn leave you weak. Sometime compromise can also be a very powerful tool. Assessing when to stand your ground and when to compromise is crucial in life.

Food for thought—What makes you stand your ground?

YOU'RE ALLOWED TO CHANGE YOUR MIND

One of the traps we encounter in life at times is this absurd idea that once we decide upon something we can never change our mind. There will always be internal and external pressure for us to commit to things. Everyone has their own opinions and ideas about pretty much everything in life. And for good reason. If we don't stick to anything, we won't ever make any progress in anything.

The problem is that we may find ourselves committing to things we hadn't intended on committing to. We might end up spending our days working toward a goal that we don't particularly believe in, but we do it because it was put in front of us. Or we felt pressured to commit to it by others. Perhaps we even fell into it because we didn't know what else to do. We all can learn what we need to do to fit into a slot that is expected of us, by grinding ourselves down into a piece that will fit. We might convince ourselves that since we've spent all this time working toward this goal that it is now important to finish it. That if we give up now, we'll never reach it despite it never being a goal that we wanted to commit to in the first place.

This is the definition of the *sunk-cost fallacy*. It is the phenomenon that happens when a person is reluctant to abandon a strategy or a course of action because they have invested heavily in it. Even when it becomes clear that abandoning it would be more beneficial for them.

When we do change our mind, and we will, it does not erase all that existed previously. We will never get the time we spent working on something back. Nor will it absolve us of any fallout that may occur from our shift in direction. We do, however, retain all the skills, memories, and lessons we learned while we were working toward that prior goal. But if you no longer believe in something, you're likely to do more damage sticking with a lie than taking the loss and moving on.

It's also important to ask yourself why you want to change your mind. Some of the most useful skills we can develop are through things that are difficult, or time consuming. Because something is difficult is a reason to stick with it. If something is difficult that means you have the most to learn from it. Challenge yourself; that's the single best way to see how far you have come, and how far you must go. Failure isn't something to fear, it's just a lesson waiting to be learned.

Thinking in extremes can be a dangerous habit, but I encourage you to think in terms of "how long do I see myself doing this for?" If it's a lifelong commitment, it will need much more serious consideration than anything that is just a temporary interest. If something only takes a month, a year then in the grand scheme of things that's a pretty low-level commitment for developing new skills to help you through life.

Food for thought—What cost are you willing to pay to change your life?

BELIEVE IN YOURSELF THE MOST

You are the reason you wake up in the morning. You are the only person in your life living your life. Throughout our life we will find people who doubt us, and people who believe in us. But at the end of the day, it comes down to believing in ourselves. No one will believe in someone who won't take up the sword to fight for their own life. We have a tough job ahead of us, for we must be both our biggest fan and our harshest critic. Every failure we have, we must analyze it and learn from it. Every success we have, we must question how we did it and move on with this new knowledge.

When we succeed, we must be our own biggest critic. When we fail, we must act as our biggest believer. Mostly, everyone else will act in the opposite manner. They will believe in us during the good times and doubt us during the bad.

What do we need the most when we are succeeding? Do we need someone who is telling us that everything we're doing is perfect and there is no room for improvement? Or do we need someone who looks at what we've done and helps us do better the next time?

What do we need more when we are hurting and when things are looking down? Do we need someone who will tell us to give up on our dreams? Someone who sees us standing on the edge and yells, "Jump?" Or do we need someone who will be there to tell us to keep our head high, that this is only temporary, and that we will rise again from the ashes like a phoenix?

Not a single person in your life has lived your life. No one knows what you have been through, the emotions you have felt, the betrayals you have suffered, or the scars you are hiding. Why would you allow them to act like they know the fire that drives you? Cherish those who are your cheerleaders during the hard times. Those individuals who even if the world turns against you, will have your back, because they are unicorns. They are mystical, and you would be a fool to hunt them for their horns.

Food for thought—How could you have done better the last time?

BE THE ONLY VALIDATION YOU NEED

If we are constantly seeking other people's validation, then we are constantly seeking others for their permission. We don't need someone else's permission to live.

But this is a lot easier said than done. Would you still do what you are doing if the world was empty? Are you putting on an act for the sake of others or are you doing it for yourself? We should strive to live every single day with intention, with confidence to know what you're doing is alright. If you wait for others to give you the green light, you'll be waiting forever. How slow would the world turn if we had to form a committee first and put to a vote what we should be doing every day?

It is important to remember that the consequences to action mirror the importance of action. There are those who act and become frightened by the waves their action created, and who recoil from even creating a ripple in the future. Then, there are those who act and choose to be ignorant of the weight of their feet. They leave a path of destruction behind them, never looking in the mirror at what they see behind them. For fear of what they would see trailing them. And there are those who act, who see the waves, and temper themselves. Instead, they use the past as an anvil, to strike their blade against. Moulding their actions so that they may walk into the future with confidence. These are people who seek to like what they see when they look at their past.

Self-validation is the ability to rely upon ourselves to act. It is the means of trusting ourselves to deal with the consequences of our own actions. It means having the confidence to trust what we are doing is the right thing. It means asking ourselves if what we are doing will cause a ripple, or a wave. Trusting ourselves with the permission to act is the very basis of our ability to survive.

Food for thought—How do you know what you're doing is right? How do you know what someone else tells you to do is right?

NOTE MORE THAN JUST THE OBVIOUS

The most interesting things in life generally don't make themselves obvious to the world. The mundane, the typical, the standard affair can be the easiest places to hide within. Many people would prefer to just live their lives, go to work every day, go home, have a warm meal, and find a place to be comfortable. They would rather live their whole life in comfort, keeping to themselves, not rocking the boat. All so that they know their next meal will be there for them.

We could just pick something to take notes on or choose something to always be paying attention to. How effective is a laser at lighting up the area around it? We would certainly notice something if we were looking for it, but we risk missing a much larger piece of the puzzle if our focus is too narrow. But we need to ask ourselves how much of our lives are we willing to dedicate to just one thing? Does the attention we pay to that one thing benefit our life enough to compensate for missing everything else?

Learning how to be observant will help us in so many ways that can't be describe with words. It's a skill that gets neglected by many because we are constantly in a rush to get from point A to point B. The easiest way to practice is to just take notes or to journal. When you see something that seems weird, that seems out of the ordinary, make a note of it. Either it will turn out to be something truly out of the ordinary, or you will realize that it is actually common place. Perhaps you just hadn't noticed it before. Either way, congratulations! You are learning how to be observant.

It's really easy to become obsessed, and to train ourselves to only see what we want to see. I want to warn against allowing yourself to become a laser. Once we start noticing things, it's hard to stop. And we're more likely to mistake one thing for another if we are always focusing on that one thing.

Remember what they say about assumptions!

Food for thought—While you are laser focused on one thing, a million missed opportunities are passing you by every day.

LIFE GOES ON—PICKING A PATH TO FOLLOW

This should be some of the most obvious advice ever provided. Somehow and sometimes the decision to do something can be intimidating. The reality is that at times it doesn't particularly matter which direction we pick, as long as it's forward. If we are learning, if we are walking down a path, we can worry about changing paths later. The only thing that we can't change is our past. Remember, although it follows us it is our past and not our future.

There's a bunch of different metaphors we can use to visualize a journey through life. Some may imagine it as a highway with thousands upon thousands of lanes. Others may think of it as dozens upon dozens of splitting paths in the woods. In either case, moving from one path to the adjacent one isn't too hard. What does tend to be difficult and maybe even dangerous is jumping suddenly from lane sixty-nine to lane four-twenty. (Granted if those were real lanes, I'd imagine there would be a shortcut between the two somewhere.)

The bigger issue about picking a direction is about the skills we will develop along the way. If we can determine what skills we would like to develop, it can then bring the paths that use those skills closer to us or easier to spot. We can let another path teach us the skills that will bring us into the future, even if we end up branching off it eventually. That is just what life is all about. The most unique thing about you is the path under your feet. So, don't get too concerned about where the path is going. Become more focused on the journey you will need take to get to where you want to end up.

Food for thought—When was the last time you came to a fork in the road?

THE ACTIONS OF OTHERS ARE IRRELEVANT

Life is complicated, but we make it harder on ourselves by comparing what we do to those around us. As we grow, you'll find some people are just parroting the words they've heard from others, but they can make it seem as if they belong to them.

Your goal is to separate what you believe from what you've heard. To judge yourself by your own actions and not the actions of others. To make the choice to walk your own path. Holding yourself accountable for your own actions means not allowing yourself to use the behaviours of others as a justification for your own. Saying it feels like it should be something that's obvious. But in practice, when you start to look around, you'll find that you're in the minority if you practise this. It is much easier to shift the blame onto others than it is to take the weight upon yourself.

There is a strength to be found here that goes unrivalled by those who do use the actions of others to judge themselves. By committing to yourself, it allows you to act freely. You will never find yourself waiting for the approval of others before you take a step. The people around you will look to step to your beat, and to match your rhythm. But do not concern yourself with them. Let them watch, let them copy you, and let them try to match how brightly you shine. Not a single person who is trying to copy you will ever surpass you in being you.

That's not to say that it is a bad thing to set a rhythm, to create a flow for those around you in which they can find comfort in. You can help people find their balance. So that they can begin to walk on their own, without having to watch your feet.

There will be times when you must steel yourself. To commit to trusting yourself that you are on the right path. You will see people around you who are achieving heights, grasping at the clouds that you wish were in your own hands. Look to others not to do as they do, but to find your own path. If you do everything that someone else does, then you will only end up living the dream of someone else.

Food for thought—Are you going to follow or are you going to lead?

TO KNOW YOUR LIMITS MEANS PUSHING YOUR LIMITS

The only way you're ever going to know what you're capable of is by seeing how far you can push yourself. To be able to know how fast you can run, you must run. To be able to run faster than your top speed, first you must run at your top speed. Some people crumble when presented with the smallest of obstacles. Some people challenge themselves so rarely that they learn to fear even the idea of failure. All a failure is, is a building block for the next part of your life. The more failures someone has under their belt, the stronger their resolve.

You could live in fear of failure, but you'll never try anything. At the end of the day, as long as you keep trying, your failures will look suspiciously like lessons. As long as you keep learning, as long as you keep putting one foot in front of the other then your progress will never stop. You won't even recognize your limits when you fly past them, as long as you keep pushing.

Some limits are easier to track than others, such as your physical limits. Physical limits are the easiest to put a number to. But your mental space has limits that you can push as well.

Let's stick to your physical limits first for your reflection.

How long can you hold your breath?

How long can you run without stopping?

How long can you stay on one task without being distracted?

Food for thought—What are the easy things you do regularly to challenge yourself?

THE END IS ONLY THE BEGINNING

If we were so fortunate, the end of all things would come quietly and the beginning of what comes next would take its place without any pause. Then none of us would even recognize that a change had occurred. However, as things stand, the change over from what came before and what will take its place can take many different forms.

No matter how destructive, how harsh an ending may feel, there will always be something that comes after. You certainly hope you will never be like one of the trees in a forest fire. But even that event makes way for new life because the ashes fertilize the ground for new life to take root.

Recognizing when something's time has come, especially when we are too close to it can be daunting. A relationship will end, and instead of allowing it to come to an end quietly, peacefully, you may find yourself clinging onto it. Simply because it's what you know, because it's comfortable, even if refusing to let go ends up killing you in the process. It's easier to see the end of something when looking in from the outside. Unfortunately, it's hard to step outside of your life to look in to make this discovery.

Your first hurdle is in accepting the state of things. You need to recognize exactly where you are in the moment, what emotions you're feeling, and acknowledge them. Your emotions could be of fear, of relief, or of anxiety. But you need to allow yourself to come to terms with those feelings. This is you feeling the flames of the fire, but this too will pass, as all things have before it.

Your second hurdle is to identify what nutrients you were left with after the fire has burned through. There may be scars, there may be blights, but you are not so weak that you must surrender to a few scrapes here and there. Ask yourself what lessons you have learned, what you have discovered about yourself in the process of living? Sometimes the growth we experience after we go through a challenge isn't obvious until our back is up against the wall.

Your final hurdle is to allow yourself to flourish from the nutrients the fire has given you. To allow new life to bloom where the old overgrown canopies once stood. Your scars are your lessons. Little reminders of the pain you went through to become the person you are now. So, don't let your suffering be for naught. Use your life as a lesson to be able to shine brighter than you ever imagined possible.

By holding onto the past and not just the lessons you learned is like you've simply attached weights onto your ankles. If you find yourself standing in a cold rainy night, feeling despair, and not knowing how to find the beginning of what comes next, you need to ask yourself these questions.

Would I go through that experience again?

What choices am I happy with?

What did I learn about myself?

If you go through life with the intention of always learning something, you will never stop moving forward.

This is what it takes to overcome a victim mindset. Not to discredit those who have been victimized. It's necessary to just be able to appreciate what comes next. And what it means to being able to move on from what came before.

Food for thought—What had to end to bring you to where you are today?

WE ALL MAKE MISTAKES

Making mistakes is part of life. Trying to live in a way that you will never make a single misstep is unrealistic. Every day we need to be walking into life greeting new opportunities and a chance to perform at our best. It is true that some of those days aren't going to go as planned. And sometimes what you think is the right thing to do will end up not being the correct choice.

Being perfect, without flaws is a fantasy, and no one should be expected to be perfect. So, forgive yourself for not being perfect.

The more you learn, the more you will realize how little you know. Just because something seems insignificant to you doesn't mean that someone else will feel the same. There will be times when you act that it will seem to be fine to your eyes, but it will appear to be a mistake in the eyes of another.

You're going to have to learn for yourself to be able to recognize the nuances here. But in general, if you intend to coexist with that person in life, it's likely easier to apologize and move on after you've been made aware that you made a mistake. You can never undo the past, so anything that you have done will always have happened. The future though is not yet decided, and it is determined by the present. No one owes you forgiveness for your missteps, and you cannot make someone forgive you. Instead, you should spend your time in the present making sure the future isn't a repeat of the past.

If you allow your mistakes to define you, you will keep making them. If you tell yourself every single day that you are a thief, a liar, and a cheat, how easy would it be for you to justify being a thief, a liar, and a cheat? You must be capable of forgiving yourself and moving past your mistakes if you intend to live in a future where you do not repeat your past mistakes.

Food for thought—What mistake are you repeating?

AN APOLOGY MEANS NOTHING WITHOUT CHANGE

It doesn't matter how many times you say you're sorry or what consequences you will face. Until you want to change yourself, you won't. Learning to forgive yourself also means learning to apologize to yourself. It means recognizing the part of you that acted. It means recognizing what impulse, or desire that led you to be there in the first place. It means recognizing where you are self-sabotaging and understanding why you did it.

It's a lot easier to know when you owe yourself an apology than when you owe someone else one. Sometimes people get upset over the weirdest things and lash out as if you should be able to read their mind. This is why a lot of apologies are issued without any meaning behind them. In the mismatch of values, if you don't believe you did anything wrong, how genuine is any apology that you have to offer? That's not to say you should change for others. If it were that easy to control people, you would see people asking for apologies for walking on the wrong side of the street!

Imagine if someone were to come up to you and demand an apology for stepping with your left foot first instead of your right. Would you ever apologize for something like that?

Instead, it would be more fruitful if someone who genuinely wants an apology were to clearly communicate their point of view first. So that you can properly understand where you went wrong and why an apology is necessary. If someone just wants to make you feel like you did something wrong, they will shy away from explaining how what you did was wrong. If they can't explain why it was wrong, then it is likely they don't even believe it themselves.

Food for thought—An unprompted apology means more than one that is asked for.

A STONE BRIDE DOESN'T BURN

Going through life you will meet countless people. Some meetings will be brief, some will stick around for a while, and some will come in and out of your life seemingly at random. There is truly little any of us can do to control the world around us beyond the actions of our two hands. A tough lesson you will have to learn is learning to accept when your connections to someone else are severed. Don't force someone to stay somewhere they don't want to be because it will just drag you down.

This is not to say that a broken bridge must stay broken. Just that once a bridge breaks, it takes both sides wanting to rebuild it for you both to rebuild it stronger and better. And it will be stronger. The foundation is in the same spot as it was before, but even if the banks of the river have gone soft, if you both are reaching out for each other then you will find somewhere that the ground feels firm. Be patient. Don't force it and have faith that if it is meant to be, it will be.

You're never going to know if the last time you speak to someone will be the last time you ever speak to them. Create friendships, love freely, care for others, but do not covet them. Accept changes that must come because when it comes your permission is not required.

Instead, build your bridges out of stone, which even the fiercest fire will leave at most temporarily impassable. Create memories, celebrate each other, catch others when they fall, and trust that those meant to withstand the test of time will do so for an eternity. All it takes is caring. Spending time with each other, making time for each other. If you want to build a strong connection with someone, then that means trying to make it happen. It also means being aware when it's one-sided; if you're the one putting in all the effort, if you're the only one reaching out, then as soon as you stop, its weakness will become apparent.

Food for thought—What bridges in your life are made of stone?

REMEMBER OTHERS FOR WHAT YOU'VE LEARNED

You are going to go through so many different experiences in life. There are going to be highs, and there will be lows. It's countless how many different people's lives you will be a part of. Some will be for a brief flash, and some will form into a much deeper connection.

When someone leaves your life, for whatever myriad of reasons, how you remember them will greatly affect your life without them. This isn't about evangelizing them or demonizing them. They always were just human, and imperfect like the rest of us. This is about holding onto what helps you grow, and holding onto the energy you want in your life.

I have no examples to offer you because the reason someone was important enough to you to make them a part of your life is up to you to decide. But not everyone sticks around and when they're gone, they are no longer a piece of your everyday life. So, how will you remember them? Did they teach you enough about yourself to deserve a place in your memory?

Or maybe it's better to ask what they learned from you? What were you to them, and what lessons will they remember you for? What part of their life were you responsible for?

Learning to recognize what you learn from others will both help you to refine yourself and to create a strong foundation with those around you. Your words carry weight. If someone is important enough to you to have earned a place in your mind, and you desire to show them gratitude, then tell them what you've learned from them.

Remember, it's a choice to be an active learner, so wear it with pride.

Food for thought—Who will you always remember?

THE PAST DOESN'T CHANGE BUT PEOPLE'S OPINIONS DO

The weirdest things happen over time, and it happens all the time. If you get too caught up in the moment, you'll find yourself being dragged along by the current. It can happen anywhere.

People will get angry about something because those around them are angry. Had you just been by yourself, separated from the rest, you may not have even felt too strongly about some perceived great injustice. It's being surrounded by voices who are louder, more prevalent that will lead you to think maybe you should feel strongly about something. This is but one of the factors that can contribute to a change in perception about past events. If only a few truly felt strongly about something, and the rest were dragged into it because they were looking for a place to belong, then how strongly do you think they will feel about it in five or ten years after it's done and settled?

Sometimes the only way we realize we were dragged into someone else's fight is when we take ourselves away from it. Being able to disengage from something and ask yourself if you are feeling your own emotions, or if you're feeling those of another. It happens all the time, and it gets the better of many of us. If you want to protect yourself from it, then just keep asking yourself why.

The other side of the equation is normalization, which can be both a poison and a cure. The more often something is done, the less anyone will care about it. The more often someone sees something, the less they will think about it. Have you ever heard someone say, "It's just the way things are." The young or the innocent are quick to make noise about something that is new to them. The old, the experienced who have seen the same thing happen repeatedly won't take any notice. Why speak up when it happens all the time?

It can be about a big deal, but it happens with small things too. If everyone decided to start wearing black and white, more people would follow suit. It happens just because it's what others are doing. It becomes "normal." All that normal is, is what we collectively have agreed upon as being normal. If it's normal to keep a notepad on you, then everyone will. If it's normal to thank the bus driver as you get off the bus, then others will too. We collectively decide what normal is.

Food for thought—What is normal now that used to be weird?

SOMETIMES THE BAD FEELINGS COME BACK

No matter how high and mighty you feel on your good days, sometimes bad feelings will sneak up on you. You'll doubt yourself; you'll question why you are even bothering to get up in the morning. You aren't any less of the person you were the day before, no matter how negative, or mean those thoughts are. They are just thoughts.

Acknowledge the thoughts. Identify what it is you're feeling. Then remind yourself that you are more than just your thoughts. It can be challenging to act in the face of negativity, and everything will feel worse while you are focused on what is wrong. The funny thing is the easiest way to get past it is to just keep on with your day. To keep moving forward, no matter what. Every day you choose to wake up, get out of bed, and continue with your life is a victory.

When you are feeling overwhelmed and when you feel like everything is too much, take a breather. Just take a moment to breathe. Count to ten and observe your surroundings.

Who can you see right now?

When did you get here?

Where are you?

Why are you here?

What are you doing right now?

This is a process called grounding, and it will help you to gain control of your surroundings.

The next step is equally as simple. Ask yourself what do you need to do next? Then, go do that.

After that step, ask yourself again, what do you need to do next? One step at a time is the only way anyone gets anything done. One foot in front of the other.

As long you keep doing that, you'll be unstoppable, no matter how much the bad thoughts tell you otherwise. As long as you can keep taking another step, then you will get to where you're going.

Food for thought—What is the next step you need to take?

DON'T HIDE BEHIND THE EXCUSES

Your greatest obstacle to your own success is you.

If you spend enough time thinking about why you shouldn't do something, then you will never do anything. If you spend enough time thinking about why something isn't you fault, then you will always be the victim.

Excuses are the complicated lies we tell ourselves why we can't do something. Excuses are telling yourself that you can't vacuum the floor because you haven't showered yet. They are used to procrastinate, or to shift blame away from you and onto some other facet that doesn't require you to act.

Aren't you better than that? Sure, there may be more to the story, but are you really completely innocent? What are you trying to achieve by shifting the blame away from you? Do you want people's pity? Do you want people to feel bad for you so they will take your side? Are you trying to pretend you're perfect? If you are asking others to take accountability for their actions, why don't you expect the same from yourself?

You may find it more helpful to practice by identifying excuses. By keeping your mind open for the times that you use an external reason to justify your behaviour. For example, I can't go for a walk, it's raining outside. The rain isn't the reason you won't go for a walk. If you wanted to, you would. Rain or not.

Food for thought—What are you avoiding taking responsibility for?

TUNE YOUR INSTINCTS

Your instincts, impulses, and desires are still powerful tools, as much as I write about avoiding giving them full control. They are tools that need tuning though, and need to be refined by life, by living each day. You are more likely to cut yourself with a dull blade than a sharp knife. Any tool you use in life should be put up for regular maintenance. Or risk when you need to rely upon it that it won't be able to do its job.

You won't find a specific way to train your instincts in this book. My lessons on instinct have all been learned through living my life and are something that no words could ever hope to replicate. However, you can still find ways to train for what matters to you. It just takes some thought about the environments you surround yourself with. There is no greater teacher than life and experiencing things first-hand.

There's over a million different jobs out there. Different positions will teach you different things, which will tune your instincts to recognize all sorts of different pieces of information. Who do you think would be better at recognizing a dangerous drunk, a CPA or a bartender? Who would be more accustomed to someone approaching them from behind, a retail worker or a police officer?

Different jobs teach a whole array of different skills, even if they aren't directly recognized. They will still train your instincts in ways that no resumé could fully explain.

Turn everything in your life into a chance to learn, and you will never stop growing. Just because the world may not recognize it, doesn't mean you haven't grown.

Food for thought—What instincts are you developing every day?

THE WORLD ISN'T EMPTY— DON'T FORCE IT

For the most part, if you push too hard on something the more likely it is to break. You may very likely find yourself in positions where you will want something to happen. Instead of being patient, instead of taking your time to proceed methodically, you will be tempted to take drastic action. The problem with drastic action or with pushing too hard on something is you're not guaranteed to like the outcome. What condition would you be in the next day if you were to spend eighteen hours at the gym in just one day? Would you be in better shape the next day after those consecutive eighteen hours in one day, or would you be in better shape by spending two and a half hours every day for a week?

There is more than one way to get the results you want. You won't avoid having to put in the effort, but the more gradually you take on something, the less pushback you will face. Hopefully, you've caught onto this by now; that consistency is everything. A little bit every day will move mountains.

Or in the case of Dashrath Manjhi, you will succeed in cutting a mountain in two.

This is just as true with people as it is with the other things in life. Consistently showing up, connecting with someone regularly is the key to building a meaningful relationship. In today's world, those who post on social media will understand this, which is why they post so regularly. To engage their viewers and to create a connection. But how real is that connection?

Instead, you should concern yourself more with consistency in your everyday life. With the people you see regularly, with the people at the grocery store, and with the people around you. You'll find friction everywhere you go, but the connections you make with another person directly cannot compare to a mirage.

Food for thought—What would you notice first? A social media friend who is not posting, or a friend you see every day who disappears.

MAKE FATE'S JOB EASIER

There is this odd middle ground between where you leave nothing to fate or trust it all to fate. You have it inside of yourself to forge ahead on whatever path you decide. Ultimately, your actions are what will determine the shape of your life. Fate is better thought of as the consequences of your actions.

As a river flows downstream, it brings along with it leaves, branches, logs, and whatever else finds its way into it. The rush of the water erodes the banks, making ways for new and diverging paths. The water will nourish the world around it as it flows, giving life to the plants and animals that feed from it. Sometimes a river flows quickly, dangerously, and sometimes it flows quietly, with ease through its world.

Your life is like that river, and all that happens on that twisting and winding path. Fate is the branches that float along with you. It's the eroding banks, which alter your course. Fate is the ocean you feed into, where all the other rivers come to merge.

Fate, however, cannot exist without your actions to feed it. And it is hungry. The bigger your actions, the more actions you take, the more drastically fate can involve itself in your life.

To put this into a modern perspective, if you make a point of saying hello to the people you see every day, one day you may find yourself in a conversation with someone. One that never would have happened had you not set the groundwork by saying hello. If a hello is too difficult, start with a wave. Start small, however small you must, but the important part is that you start.

Food for thought—Who is the next person you will say hello to?

Hello. Bonjour. Hola. Pryvit. Nǐn hǎo. Salve. Konnichiwa. Guten. Tag Olá. Anyoung haseyo. Asalaam alaikum. Goddag. Shikamoo. Goedendag. Yassas. Dzień dobry. Selamat siang. Namaste, Namaskar. Merhaba. Shalom. God dag.

If you like how a language sounds, learn to speak it.

Thank You. Merci. Gracias. Dyakuyu. Xiè xiè. Grazie. Arigatou. Danke. Obrigado. Gahm-sa-ham-ni-da. Šukran. Tak. Asante. Bedankt. Sas efharistó! Stokrotne dzięki. Anda sungguh baik hati. Dhanyavaad. Teşekkür ederim. Toda. Tack själv. Takk skal du ha.

LOVE YOURSELF FIRST

This may sound like an obvious piece of advice when it is said out loud, but how many times have you tried to push away your own self-doubt, your own self-hatred along with the affection of others? How many times have you done something for someone else because you thought it would make them or those around you like you? How broken and shattered is your cup that you try to fill it with the cups of others?

The irony is that the only way you can really help others in any meaningful way is after you have found a way to help yourself first. It's as they say, "a rising tide lifts all boats," but the opposite also rings true. If you are falling, unless those around you have the strength, you risk bringing all those around you down with you. In this way each of us is Atlas, carrying the weight of the world on our shoulders.

So, fix the cracks in your cup. Glue the pieces back together and fill it so that it overflows into the cups of those around you without any added effort on your part. What more could you ever ask for than to have the strength to lift others by lifting yourself?

If you are going to love yourself, you need to take care of yourself. And if you're not used to it, it can be very daunting. Even basic tasks can be excruciating to stick with. You will convince yourself it's not worth it. You will tell yourself there is no point. Sure, the reward for living is death, as it comes for all of us, but would you choose to wait for it silently or face it head-on?

I offer this suggestion. Growing up or growth is about going from being carried by others, to carrying yourself, and to carrying others. There is no greater accomplishment than when the people you've helped achieve their dreams. If life is but a game, then play it as such.

You can't will yourself to love yourself. You must work toward it. Don't let all your hard work go to waste.

Food for thought—Are you neglecting your self-care? Your hygiene, your sleep, and your diet are all part of loving yourself.

YOU DON'T HAVE TO BE ALONE

One of the many contradictions you will face throughout life is the idea that you need to be totally self-sufficient, not relying on others, and trusting only yourself. In practice this is much harder said then done, and for *most* people completely unnecessary. No matter how capable you are as an individual, your actions are only that of one person. So, becoming self-reliant and trusting yourself is only the first step in contributing to the community.

In the process of growing up, we go from being babies, who are fully dependant on the outside world to provide us with all our needs, to functioning adults who can meet, and eventually exceed our own needs. Somewhere along the line some of us get addicted to the feeling of individualism, to only being responsible for ourselves, and we retreat away from others in fear of surrendering the peace that we have found. There lies a danger in taking too much pride in one's own abilities, because without the humility to recognize when you need help you risk drowning yourself when no one is looking.

The best relationships, the best friendships, the best places you will find that fit you are the ones that you can enter and exit with ease. If you think of yourself as a puzzle piece, then you can find the people that your piece slides into gracefully.

Some friction is always expected, but you shouldn't have to sand your edges down just to fit in somewhere you don't want to be.

Food for thought—Independence can be lonely, but dependence can be suffocating. How do you find the right balance?

TALKING TO PEOPLE

We are fed this crazy notion that talking to people, hearing what others have to say is scary. That by talking to someone you will put yourself at risk. To a degree that's true. By talking to people, you will be introduced to different people with different world views. This simple act of learning about different ways of life will kill the person you were before and replace you with someone who sees others not as a source of fear, but a source of knowledge.

A question for the would-be protagonists out there. When playing a video game, do you speak to only the highlighted quest givers? Or do you speak to the townsfolk, looking for what additional information you can find? Do you ever look to learn about something hidden, or perhaps find side quests by treading off the beaten path?

Talking to people really doesn't have to be such a terrifying endeavour. It just takes some practice, especially if you're used to talking over social media. By the very nature of it, communicating digitally makes conversations more transactional and less personal. It's easy to forget that the person talking to you is a living, breathing person, or possibly not even that when we rely exclusively on digital communication.

The important part to never forget is that each person you talk to has their own priorities. And much like in video games, they may not have anything to say to you. Some people will only talk to you in certain locations. Or if you're after certain information, you will need to meet certain criteria for them to speak to you.

Food for thought—It's not the world's job to orient itself around you, nor is it on you to orient yourself around the world. How do you find people to talk to and find things in common with them?

MOST PEOPLE JUST WANT TO BE HAPPY

The unfortunate reality we live in is it's hard to know who we can trust. Everyone has different motivations for their actions, and everyone has allegiances to different places and people. Everyone has a different opinion about what will bring them happiness. What is common is that just about everyone wants to be happy.

Trust is one of those things that you must build over time, and you may inherently start with a base level among some people, but with others you must work toward it. There is nothing wrong with treating others with kindness along with a base level of respect. This will go a long way in establishing a relationship between you and someone whose trust you seek. At the end of the day, the motivations, and the allegiances don't matter as much between two people who trust each other.

In your quest to learn from others, to gain the trust and co-operation of those around you, and your larger quest of finding what makes you personally happy, you may find yourself doing things to make others happy. You must be careful playing that game.

At most we can offer someone a crutch to aid them in finding their balance. And you may find yourself seeking to make others happy at the expense of your own happiness. The most anyone can offer another person to make them happy is a temporary experience, a distraction, or a dopamine high. It can't be bottled and sold no matter how often we are told, "This will make you happy."

There is nothing wrong with living your life in the service of making others happy, or in offering a crutch to those in need. Those in need can sometimes become too reliant on that crutch, convincing themselves they cannot stand without it. It's crucial that you don't place yourself in that position. Holding someone's hand while travelling over a hill is a much different story than carrying them on your back. It's important to review your intentions, making sure what you are doing isn't hurting you, or those you are trying to help.

You will come up with any excuse you can to justify helping someone who is important to you. And by no means am I advocating for you not to help. We all need help from time to time, a hand to hold, or a light in the dark.

What I am advocating for is to think twice about how you can help. The age-old saying goes, "Give a man a fish, you feed him for a day; Teach a man to fish, you feed him for a lifetime." Sometimes all we can offer to someone is a fish, but if you have the capability of teaching someone to fish, then their entire life will be more abundant.

The same goes for the illusive state of happiness. Are you offering a fish, or are you offering to teach them to fish? Whatever form the aid you offer takes, it remains true that everyone wants to be happy. Finding a way to help someone achieve that state can help you to form a connection with those people. What you can do to help really depends upon who you are as a person, and what each person can offer someone else is unique to them. You can take inspiration from others to find what fits you the best. To help you find your own happiness.

We are sold on the idea that if you just get this next thing, this next achievement, pass this next hurdle that it will make you happy. It may, for a time. Completing things feels good, seeing what you've learned, and the talents you've developed through reaching your goal is not something to scoff at. But that feeling won't last, and then you will move onto the next thing that you think will give you happiness.

Food for thought—You are never going to find happiness if you are always demanding others to give it to you. What relationship do you think taking care of yourself, and loving yourself has with being happy?

EVERYONE'S HEART BEATS

You need to drive it home in your thoughts that every single person you meet has a life outside of your own. Every single one of them has friends and family doing their own things, living their own lives. The person you briefly walked by was born and grew up around completely different people than you. They have been hurt, have been healed, and have been hurt again. Likely they've loved, and they've hated. They might be living the best moment of their life, or they might have just suffered a loss that there are no words to express. You might never cross paths with that person again. You'll never know what's happening in their life, but it will still happen. Life never stops. That's the one constant you can rely on.

C'est la vie.

The reason the butterfly effect is so terrifyingly beautiful is because of that one pure, undeniable fact. If you help someone, and your help lets them go on to help someone else, then the chain will never end.

But it's a sharp blade, and both sides can cut. If you hurt someone, you have no way of knowing who else you'll hurt down the road. A careless cigarette butt can start wildfires, which burn the homes of wild things, both human and not.

Kindness has the best return on your investment. It costs nothing, and it radiates to each person it touches.

Food for thought—What kindness can you offer every day?

CURATE YOUR WORLD

The easiest thing you can do to change your life is to change what is in your life. Drastic changes can be rough and leave scars, whereas it can take time to see the influence of small changes. The small things are simple things that often get overlooked. Your diet is not simply what you eat, it's what you consume, what you pay attention to, who you spend time with, and the music you listen to.

It's a lot easier said than done, and to make room for change you must be willing to put aside what already takes up that space. That is not a decision that should made lightly, and it will likely weigh on you even after you've made it. It would be foolish to suggest one way of life is better than another, so don't think you should make changes just for the sake of change. The decisions you make for your life should be made for the sake of your life.

If you only act in the interest of others, you will only ever benefit others. If you only change your life because someone told you to, then that change will be temporary at most. You must want to change your life if you want to see any substantial change appear and become a significant part of your life.

This sounds like a much bigger task than it really is. You can start small, such as not watching things you don't like. If you don't like horror movies, don't watch them. It doesn't mean they don't exist, but life is too short to spend your leisure time doing things you don't like. If the people you are spending time with are doing things you don't want to participate in, then stop spending time with them. Find people who have interests in common with you.

Life is that simple. Participate in what you enjoy, distance yourself from what you don't.

Food for thought—What things are you participating in that you don't like? Why are you engaging in these activities?

ACKNOWLEDGE YOUR FAULTS AND INNER DEMONS

It's really easy to refuse anything that you can't perceive, so acknowledging what an emotion feels like, or recognizing an impulse that physically exists will be harder for some than others. To satisfy that little part of you that can't take things on faith, when you give into an impulse, or are feeling emotions, there are chemicals being released in your brain. Chief among them is dopamine. Boiled right down, your actions are to satisfy your brain's drug addiction.

In comes the seven deadly sins. On their own in small doses they are just people giving into their impulses. If you're going to fault someone for giving into theirs, make sure to look in the mirror to see where you are giving into yours. The sins just function as a convenient way to personify the various ways our body encourages us to act. Once you can identify and recognize a feeling, it is easier for you to act against it. This is the same as everything in nature, just applied to the illusive "feelings."

The cost of giving into these impulses, of allowing them to control your life is, well, if I was religious, I'd say your eternal soul. Keeping our focus on the real world, giving into your impulses just drives you further and further into addiction. The more you give in, the more you will need to reach that same feeling. You will find you start to organize all your decisions around satisfying that feeling.

Impulses on their own aren't bad; a lot of them are there to keep you alive. It's the same thing as "all things in moderation." If you always give in to an impulse, then it is harder to deny it when it comes calling. Some impulses though will actively harm you, and sometimes we even know it's bad for us, but we keep doing it anyways. Just start with recognizing them, then worry about controlling them.

Food for thought—How are you hurting yourself?

GREED JUST MEANS MONEY, RIGHT

Stop me if you've heard this one before.

Don't be greedy.

Take only what you need.

Pigs get slaughtered.

Greed will distort your vision. You'll see gold where none exists. You'll think the world is owed to you, and you'll be fooled into thinking the world exists for you.

Greed teams up with sloth to lead you into thinking that if you just wait long enough something will change. It would have you trusting your fate to luck. How long would you spend every day doing the same thing expecting change? How long are you going to lay in bed wondering when things will "get better?" Change happens for those who take action to make it happen.

Greed and envy will encourage you to covet another person's success, as if what someone else has belongs to you. You'll pay no heed to the work they have put in to achieve their goal. Instead, you will focus solely on why you deserve their life more than they do. You only have your life; wouldn't you rather build a life tailor-made for you instead of the life of another?

Overall, the pitfalls that greed will offer to you are those of shortcuts, surefire low effort paths. It will entice you to keep taking everything you can, and you'll leave the world around you with nothing. You'll push everyone away with your greed, starving them to fill your coffers. But you'll never have enough.

Food for thought—What is too much?

THE SLOTH GETS A BAD REP

Much like the animal, the sin of sloth moves slowly, with purpose. It will creep into every aspect of your life if you allow it, acting as weights, and making everything you do more taxing. The more you allow yourself to be slothful, the more it will weigh you down. The more often you allow yourself to be lazy, to take shortcuts, to push things off until later, the more you will be tempted to act like this.

It will cling to you like a vine, draining away everything about you. Your dreams will seem to be an impossible climb. You will fall into excuses to put off what needs to be done. Everything will require effort and making that effort will be less and less enticing. You'll stop appreciating that there are rewards for your efforts. You'll turn into a husk, without any substance. You will expend so little energy, but never have any energy to spare.

Sloth will destroy your entire life; you won't even realize how deep you've dug your hole by the time you do look up. It may seem to be one of the lesser sins, disguising itself as rest, but its cruelty will leave you with nothing.

Holding yourself accountable to your actions, even simply acting is a step against falling for its tricks. Like everything we've talked about up to this point, be an action taker, and take pride in the effort it takes to achieve things. Take in what you learn while you do the work. Effort isn't something that should be avoided.

Rest is important. Its influence will always be there, but do not trust it with your life, because it will devour your dreams while you lay dreaming of a better life.

Food for thought—What are you avoiding putting effort into?

ENVY FOR A LIFE THAT IS NOT YOURS

It can be tricky to pin envy down, and to recognize it when it comes to call. It's an ugly feeling that if allowed to run rampant will create feelings of inferiority. It will feed into a resentment of others, even if those others harbour no ill will toward you. In this way it will bind your hands and blind your eyes. It will encourage you to place all your misfortune onto the circumstances beyond your control.

If you allow it to run rampant in your mind, you will spend all your time comparing yourself to others, living to their standards, and not on raising your own.

Which of these two examples do you think will make it harder to live your life.

Person A is striving for someone else's goal. They set their sights on what other's have and want their life, their relationships, and their success.

Person B is striving to improve themself for their own sake. They allow whatever is to come and to enter their life.

How much energy do you think someone who chooses option B spends on thinking about someone who picked option A?

Are you living the life of person A or are you person B?

You're never going to have someone else's parents. You're never going to have a chance to grow up in a different way, no matter how much you wish it. The past will never change. All you have control over is right here and now.

Especially when things feel like they aren't going well, don't waste your precious energy on worrying about what is going well for someone else. Use your energy on your life, worry about making each day a little bit better, piece by piece. Incremental consistent growth will change your life.

Food for thought—Who are you comparing yourself to?

A SLAVE TO LUST

How quiet our world would be if no one ever gave into their lust. We may be smart enough to plan ahead for multiple winters, but we never stop being animals. Our desires, our impulses help to keep us alive, and that includes living on as a species. Sometimes I worry we forget to care about the wild animal on the inside. The part of us that doesn't think, that reacts, that gets scared when there is a loud noise. The part of us that craves the accompaniment of others.

Surrendering themself to lust, however, is sure to have been the end of some people in the past ages. Too many mouths to feed isn't exactly a new problem, and before modern science got involved that was a common way by which lust stole from its victims.

The miracle of modern science seemingly has conquered any obstacle of our indulging in our earthly desires. And as free of repercussions as possible. Though, it could be argued we've never been more consumed by lust than when it appears to be consequence free.

It's not wrong to want something or someone. In fact, it's completely natural, and it's how we are all here today. The danger of wanting comes when it turns into an obsession. When you lose your ability to control yourself. When that happens, you'll end up causing damage that you'd otherwise have never caused.

Someone who's surrendered to lust will be led by it. The danger isn't in finding your spouse attractive, but by basing all your decisions around that feeling. By being easily swayed by another. By giving into impulse when given the opportunity. Lust will still steal your life, though these days it looks less like too many mouths to feed, and more like being in situations that you will come to regret.

Food for thought—Wanting is not bad. Acting without thought is what can be dangerous.

TAKE PRIDE IN BEING HUMBLE

Taking pride in one's work and in one's self is important. What you achieve is important to you. No one can take the work you've done on yourself away from you and having pride in that work is important.

Where pride becomes dangerous is in its way of making you think that you're done. That your last accomplishment will always be your last. That because of who you are, you don't need to take any more action. Pride will blind you from seeing you need to act by inflating what you've done beyond its scope. Pride will make you too proud to see the cracks in your work. You can fall victim to thinking that you are infallible. There's always more to do.

No matter how great you think you are, you are but one person, one life, and one voice. Your time on this planet is a tiny blip in comparison to the entire history of humans, and in terms of what has come to pass, and what is yet to come. Even the greatest accomplishments of our lives will turn to sand as the hourglass keeps turning.

Do not despair for your life, as it is yours to live. It may not be the most important in comparison to the rest of history, but its importance to you is at the apex. Your life is more important to you than anything else the world has to offer, no matter how big or small you are. Take pride in what you do but be humbled by how small you are. If you allow pride to walk freely over your life, you will limit yourself to only what you've already done, and not what you can still do.

Pride will devour your future while you are stuck reminiscing about your past glory.

Food for thought—If you're done, what's next?

GLUTTONY EXISTS EVERYWHERE

We've all heard it haven't we? The phrase of being a glutton for punishment.

You might not even realize you're doing it, but you're going to find that you do things to punish yourself. And likely for things that don't matter. Gluttony is not reserved to pigging out on snacks. It's much sneakier than that, and you'll bring it onto yourself.

It can take the form of self-sabotage or of self-harm. It comes over you as self-hatred incarnated. Whether it is brought on by a lack of self-worth, or guilt for some perceived or actual wrongs you have inflicted. It is at these times where you do something that just makes things harder for yourself. It's the acts that you do, which you expect to be punished for. Daring the world to tell you that you're wrong.

It is also the constant need for more, the endless insatiable hunger for another one. It is not limited to another cookie. It can take the form of another episode of your latest show, or another video game even if you have several that you have yet to even start. Gluttony is the endless consumption of everything: pain, pleasure, and poison. It will consume you and convince you that you're living like a king while your body and mind deteriorates into paste.

Food for thought—What feels like you can never have enough of?

THERE IS ALWAYS SOMEONE WITH MORE WRATH

It's unlikely that any of the other sins can match the malice and rage that spawns from allowing wrath to have its way. It's one of those things that spawns more of itself in others, creating an endless cycle. Any satisfaction you may find from giving into its allure will be short lived. No matter how someone has wronged you, the wrathful approach will be brief, explosive, and carry a heavy cost.

There is a very useful lesson that anyone who has learned self-defence can attest to when dealing with wrath. It can just as easily be applied to your internal battles as well as your external ones. It is easier to redirect or deflect than it is to stop. To rephrase that statement, use your opponent's momentum against them.

Find an outlet for the energy and you'll find it easier to manage. If you find yourself in its grasp, take yourself away, and release the energy. Even if someone has wronged you, you can do more with a level head than you can in that moment. Allowing wrath to reign over your actions would be the equivalent of inviting the wrath of others onto you. Think of the most heinous, grotesque act that you would commit in the name of wrath and know that you are inviting that to be done to you if you allow it to control your life.

Food for thought—What anger are you holding onto and how can you let it go?

BY THE TIME YOU'RE DESPERATE YOU'RE ALREADY LOSING

Desperation is dangerous because it can lead people to do things that they would never do otherwise. You'd think that it would take a lot for some people to become desperate, but the scale is all over the place. Some people will convince themselves there is no alternative to justify their desperate actions. Some will push themselves into desperation so that they do not have an alternative course of action. Some people are forced into it by the world around them. No matter where you fall, by the time you are at a point where "you will do anything" it's too late to have another choice.

Survival comes first, and if you must act to stay alive, then stay alive. But desperation is only that, survival. It's pushing someone else under the water so that you can breathe. It's setting fire to your house so that you don't freeze in the night. No matter what brought you to it, don't treat the willingness to do anything lightly.

Often, one of the biggest strengths you can have is understanding what you are not willing to do. By placing restrictions on yourself, you gain a better idea of what you are capable of. Sometimes you just can't see an answer that is staring you straight in the face because you are too preoccupied thinking about the one that is consuming your thoughts. This is how people lead themselves into desperation. There may be other options, but they've blinded themselves to them.

Desperation won't allow you to thrive. At most it will feed you for a day, and possibly leave you even worse off than you were the day before. If you must act to survive, find a way that builds for tomorrow, not that sacrifices your tomorrows.

Addiction kills in more ways than one.
There are more things to get addicted to in this world than you could ever imagine. And even more when you recognize that addiction isn't limited to just substances. The phrase "all things in moderation" never stops being true. Life as we know it needs water to live, and even that requires moderation.

No matter where you are in life, chances are you will face some form of addiction a couple of times in your life.

The typical dangers take the form of substances, from something as innocent as sugar to something as deadly as illicit compounds. These things prey on you to consume more to achieve an equivalent feeling.

Those who have yet to struggle against a substance addiction can't imagine what it's like when someone says, "You always need more." Should you find yourself blessed with never having experienced that state, I'll do my best to explain it to you in a way that hopefully encourages you to never feel the need to, or if you do, to be able to stop yourself.

It's a lot easier to start, than it is to stop.

At the core, our body's natural ability is to build resistance to things it is exposed to. This can turn addiction into the dangerous form of "chasing the dragon." That first time is the most dangerous, because it will set itself up for unrealistic expectations. The same dose you had before won't give you the same feeling. So, you'll justify it with, "I'll just have a bit more; it won't hurt." How many times are you willing to say, "One more can't hurt." If we're talking about something as innocent as cookies, how long before you eat an entire box of them? It might seem ludicrous to compare a dangerous substance to cookies, but if it no longer seems dangerous to you, is there a difference?

That's just the way that addiction kills and that everyone knows about it already.

Once you start liking it, once it is something that you find yourself going back to regularly, you will always find excuses to get it. Before you tried it, how often did you think about it? Likely the answer is almost never, but after you do, that answer changes. You might tell yourself you don't "need" it, but how often are you using it?

How many cigarette smokers have you met that say they can quit at anytime but still smoke at least one a day, every day? How often do you think they thought about going outside for a smoke before they started?

One of the problems with addiction is it becomes this thing that worms its way into your brain and holds your thoughts hostage. Where once upon a time you could focus on writing a paper for four hours straight, now you find excuses to "take a smoke break." It breaks up your thoughts, and it takes away from the rest of your life to satisfy a craving that ultimately poisons you.

Your life starts to revolve around filling that craving. Your decisions, which once were focused on building your life are now centred on how to refill your supply. You will start changing your habits to fulfill a need that you didn't have before. Devoting your life to something that pays no heed to your well being. Addiction becomes this all-encompassing thing where you would spend hours upon hours each day to fill it.

If there is someone reading this who is in the middle of their struggle with addiction, are you happy with how much of your life is devoted to it? How many hours of your days are spent on it? If you spent that same amount of time working out each day, what kind of shape would you be in?

Addiction will kill you because your life stops being about you.

Food for thought—What are your dependencies? What can you not go without?

AND INTO THE FUTURE WE RIDE– BE DELIBERATE OR DON'T

Picking and choosing the actions we take, what we think is best can be a chore. Making the conscious decision to act, and to know why we decide to put ourselves into specific places is important for controlling how we live our life. That is, if you want time it will continue on regardless. Finding a middle ground between constant conscious acts and trusting your instincts seems to be what many of us are after.

Wouldn't it be better to trust your instincts? To be able to know that even if you aren't making a conscious decision, that the decision you are making is in the best interest of your future? Be deliberate in your choice to act and be deliberate in your choice of trusting yourself to act.

Can you trust yourself to be ready when you need to be ready? We're all just acting on tiny fragments of information, through what we've heard from others, and from our perception of the truth.

When you can't have complete information, can you trust yourself to act when you're met with silence? There will be times in your life when you want nothing more than to be told what to do, and how to do it. As if by surrendering yourself to the will of others will alleviate you of the burden of thought. If you are feeling this way, that you have no idea how to take the next step forward, what will you do if no one tells you what that next step is? Will you step forward regardless into the dark with confidence?

Food for thought—How long would you sit and wait before you decide to be deliberate in your actions?

SYMBOLISMS OF LIFE

The world is awash with symbolism, both conscious and unconscious. Some will adopt symbols into their lives without even realizing what those symbols represent. In some of these cases their self-conscious will tell on them for choosing a symbol they feel connected to, without knowing what that symbol represents.

A million different movements could be made under the same symbol. If each little bubble never spoke to one another, they would all believe the symbol belonged to them and their movement. You could spend your life avoiding symbols, to not be counted as part of any of it. But before you know it, you might turn yourself into a symbol in the process. The weirdest thing about a symbol is it can mean different things to different observers.

Symbolism is everywhere. We create symbols out of even the most ordinary things. Sometimes we are unified in the meaning they convey, and sometimes we create our own meaning attached to them. If we allow them, they will evolve with us. They likely won't impact your day-to-day life, but they will inevitably be part of it in some form or another.

If the clothes someone wears represent a movement, does every single person wearing those clothes represent that movement? It would seem far more likely that some would wear the clothing they choose to wear simply because it's what they enjoy, and not because it holds a deeper meaning. To further this point, the clothes we wear also can act like the feathers of a peacock. If someone chooses to match what another wears, are they doing so to attract someone who matches them?

The danger of symbolism lies in the lack of communication. They can convey an intention discreetly; however, they also are in danger of miscommunication. They can cause difficulty in making sure the intended message is received. A symbol can represent a greater whole, but, symbols are also just a single piece or object that without meaning is nothing. They are only as powerful as we make them. Just because a symbol means something deep and emotional to one person doesn't mean another person will even notice it. This is how they are both dangerous, and harmless.

Food for thought—What symbolism do you recognize?

THE MATCH AND MIRROR, AND OUR FEATHERS

One of the most universal, basic subconscious acts we put ourselves through is that of finding a partner. We'll try so many different things to attract a person to us, to make things feel familiar, and yet exciting. Without familiarity we would find it hard to trust, to open our hearts up to possible pain. Without a sense of wonder, without something exciting, something to learn, we would lack the desire to seek companionship.

Our clothes, our hair, our shoes, and our appearance. They are our feathers. They are the first thing anyone sees about us. Whether someone chooses to approach us or not will largely depend on their opinion of the feathers that we wear. If we feel someone is dangerous, if the feathers they wear are intimidating, we may act wary of them. However, this is also where we might mirror their feathers.

If we choose to be similar, to create a sense of familiarity it will bridge the gap between us.

While we're young, when we are thrown together in tight places and made to talk to one another, approaching another person is forced. As we age, we bring with us our pain, our betrayals, and our life that we've lived up to that point. Our feathers may be bright, but we're cautious of a poisonous bite.

The match and mirror act only as the initial opening. They make approaching an otherwise unapproachable person easier. There's always the game of love to be played. The touch and go, the quick glance in the crowd, eye contact on a dark night are about trying to create a connection. Even if it is only a few feet once every couple of months, it may feel as though all of space and time separate you.

If there exists something you desire, your actions should reflect that. Don't expect fate to find you hidden away in a dark room. If you want fate to act, you must act first.

Food for thought—What would it take for you to approach someone you don't know?

THERE'S MORE THAN ONE GAME BEING PLAYED

For all the questions that are asked about the nature of our world, both those based in fiction and nonfiction seem to be asked from the position that the nature of our world absolves us of the consequences of our actions. What great fools we are to think that the world will just reset, as if we intend to just surrender and give up living.

Suppose for even a moment, that this world is a simulation. Even if that were the case, this would be a more complicated simulation than anything we could even fathom building. Even if it were a fantasy world, some great being's creation, some dream world, the pain we all feel is real. When we go to sleep at night, the actions of yesterday continue to ring through to tomorrow.

Even if this world means nothing to anyone outside of it, it's our world. And it's real to us.

The games being played throughout the world are endless. How you choose to live your life depends upon your actions. It's not that life imitates games, it's that games imitate life.

Every single person you see is playing their own version of this ridiculous game we call life. Sometimes we get dragged into the games of another person, and sometimes we drag others into ours. At the end of the day, each person has their own motivations, and to treat them as anything less would be to underestimate someone.

Food for thought—What has your attention?

AVOID THE SPOTLIGHT—THE GAME

Considering how dangerous being the centre of attention is, it's amazing how desperately some seek to taste its warmth. It would probably be better thought of as a game of hot potato, where the only winning move is not to play.

Once you start playing, you're playing for life. You'll be dodging its gaze everywhere you go, allowing it to shine onto someone who thinks they want it.

What are the dangers of catching the spotlight, you ask?

That depends on who you are.

What would happen if people you didn't know started listening to you?

What would happen if people you didn't know knew where you lived?

What would happen if people you didn't know asked about you from your family and friends?

What would happen if people you didn't know formed opinions about you without ever spending time with you?

The spotlight can be a blessing, but just as the sun can leave you burned, so too can spending too much time under the spotlight.

Food for thought—A sense of caution will do you wonders. Why do you think I suggest caution?

SOME WOUNDS TAKE LONGER TO HEAL

At least with physical wounds they do us the honour of being visible. People understand and can see we are hurt. When they are healed, they stay healed. We're not as lucky with emotional wounds, although I'm sure some neuroscience nerds could tell us what traumatic emotional damage does to the connections within our brain.

At least with physical wounds, after the bleeding has stopped, and it's scabbed over we can still tell it's not fully healed. But we're not as lucky with our emotional wounds. We can be going through life, trying to find a semblance of normal, a semblance of balance. And we may not realize that we've scraped the emotional wound, and it has started to bleed again. Plus, it is not as evident to others that we are wounded.

Some wounds cut so deep that you are changed for life. You heal from it, and you learn to withstand the pain before you learn to forget about the pain. But you don't tend to forget that you were wounded in the first place.

But after all, all they are is wounds and they will heal. You'll learn something from them, and life will continue marching on. If it's not fatal, are you going to pretend like it is? There's nothing wrong with using your experience to temper your actions, to keep yourself safe from danger, but you will risk giving up smiling if you always remain on high alert in your life. Accept the fact you were hurt but keep moving forward toward your goal and a better life.

Food for thought—What wound of yours needs a little more time to heal?

KEEP PRACTISING

Practice. It's the one thing you can always do to keep growing, to always be putting one foot in front of the other.

Practice saying hello.
Practice standing on one leg.
Practice drawing a circle.
Practice asking how you are feeling.
Practice counting.
Practice jumping.
Practice holding your breath.
Practice listening to others.
Practice making choices.
Practice saying no.
Practice saying yes.
Practice making breakfast.
Practice sleeping in.
Practice relaxing.
Practice swimming.

Practice running.
Practice writing your thoughts.
Practice being decisive.
Practice falling.
Practice getting back up.
Practice telling the truth.
Practice kindness.
Practice forgiving.
Practice apologizing.
Practice being the person you want to be.
Practice everything.
Practice living.
Practice saying, "I Love You."

Practice is what keeps you moving forward. Practice is what can help you find your passion and goals.

Food for thought—What are you bad at? Some practice will change that.

RELAX—DON'T TAKE IT TOO SERIOUSLY

Alright, alright, alright. I've said a lot of words to fill your head full of questions. Here's comes the part I must remind you about. Take a deep breath. Exhale.

Relax.

There are people everywhere who spend their entire lives watching their backs. There are people everywhere who tiptoe through life so that they may arrive safely at death.

Life is serious. The pain we feel is real, and our lives are full of loss. They are also full of love, full of friends, full of new experiences, and full of growth. Don't spend your life only looking at the darker parts of life. If you do, that is all you will see.

But you must remember to take a step back occasionally, to let life be what it will be. Trust that the work you will do and have done will provide for you. Trust that life will happen. You will cry because you're sad, and for reasons of joy.

Take a deep breath. Exhale.

Why are you taking everything so seriously? Do you intend to live until the sun expands and engulfs the earth? Humanity has only been recording history for roughly five thousand years, and what percentage of that time makes up your life?

Food for thought—Are you spending more time worrying about what hasn't happened yet than what you need to do next?

DON'T AIM FOR PERFECTION

Perfection is this weird unattainable goal that each and everyone of us has a different opinion about. Perfect in the eyes of the world would surrender all that it means to be human. Could you live your life free from ever making mistakes?

Perfection is just a trap to convince us that we aren't good enough as we are. Your life is beautiful because it is your life, and don't let someone else tell you that you are worth less. Calling someone else perfect would be to ask them to never change. To stay exactly as they are. Why would you curse someone with that existence?

The flaws in someone are what give people depth, and they are what makes up who someone is. Would this world really be better if everyone was just a clone of one another? It might be more organized, and it might be easier to treat it like a computer system. One where each piece fits nicely with the pieces next to it. Is the goal of humanity really to see how closely we can mimic a machine?

Life can be messy. Things change. Lives get changed by the actions of others, and it never stops. No matter how clean, how organized you try to be, sometimes things fall apart. The only person living your life is you, so don't spend it romanticizing something as cruel and deceptive as "perfection."

Food for thought—What did you last agonize over because it wasn't "perfect?"

THE FUTURE IS BLINDING

Planning for the future is a great skill. Being able to look ahead and figure out what you need to achieve the goals you have. It can be dangerous though if you spend too long thinking about what is yet to come. If you do, you can lose track of your feet. Not only that, but while you're busy worrying about what you will need to do tomorrow, it will take away from what needs to be done today. The future will come whether you want it to or not. What determines how you will walk into it is what you do in the present.

There's an ebb and flow to the world, much like the tides of the ocean. They will rise, and they will fall, before they inevitably rise again. Watching the tides is important. Some crossings are impassable at low tide, and if you aren't careful, you'll find yourself beached waiting for the tides to rise again. So, it becomes equally as important to watch your course and adjust it for the changing of the tides.

Our futures have always been intertwined; our ripples in the world playing off each other. Only now, I've introduced myself to you. How will you respond to my call to act and take ownership of your life?

ABOUT THE AUTHOR

Be the leader you would follow.

Thomas acknowledges and respects the ləkʷəŋən people on whose traditional territory he grew up on, and the Songhees, Esquimalt, and W̱SÁNEĆ people whose historical relationships with the land continue to this day.

Thomas has lived a relatively low-key life. Generally keeping to himself, he tends to avoid large public gatherings as they can be exhausting. He's always been a big fan of the question "why?" Asking it of the world around him, and more importantly, asking it of himself.

That the powerful play goes on, and you may contribute a verse.

Walt Whitman, O Me! O Life! 1892

Manufactured by Amazon.ca
Acheson, AB